Celebrating Syed

Independent in functional use

Created by Luke Thompson

Co-author Caroline Bennett

Illustrated by Kat Willott

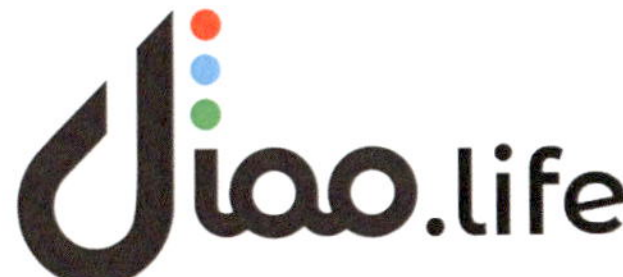

Published by Jiao Ltd
Jiao.life

Scan the QR codes to access the digital book or listen to the audio book.

Audiobook

Digital Book

The Seven Stages of Switch Development

Celebrating Syed is part of the Switch Heroes, social stories created to support switch-users with their Switch progression. The Switch Heroes series is part of the Seven Stages of Switch Development, created by Occupational Therapist and AT specialist Luke Thompson.

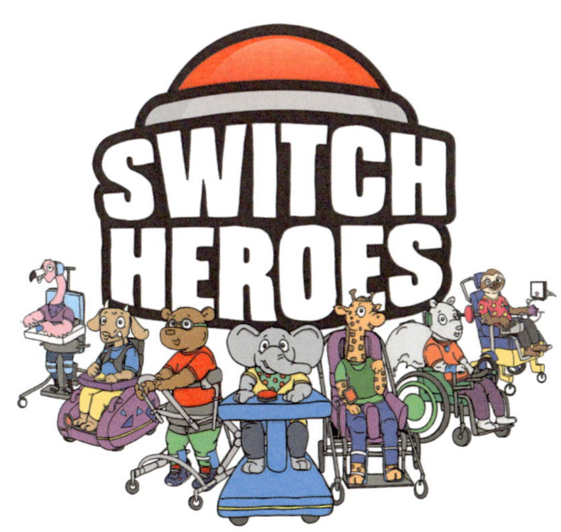

We’re celebrating Syed

Like we’ll be celebrating you!

For using your switches
so brilliantly

For all the things you want to do

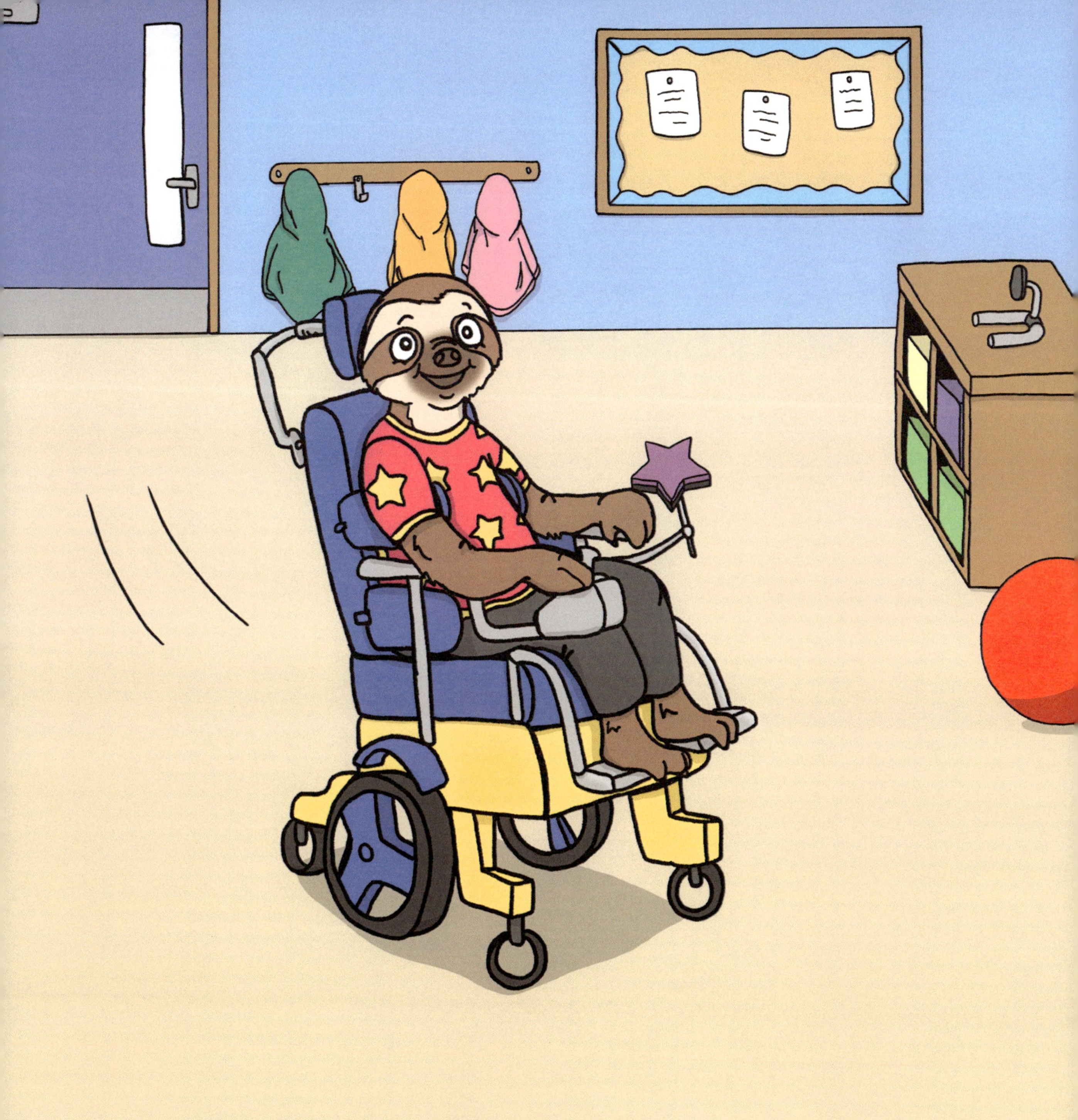

Syed is in his classroom

Enjoying morning break

Playing his computer game

Seeing what he can make

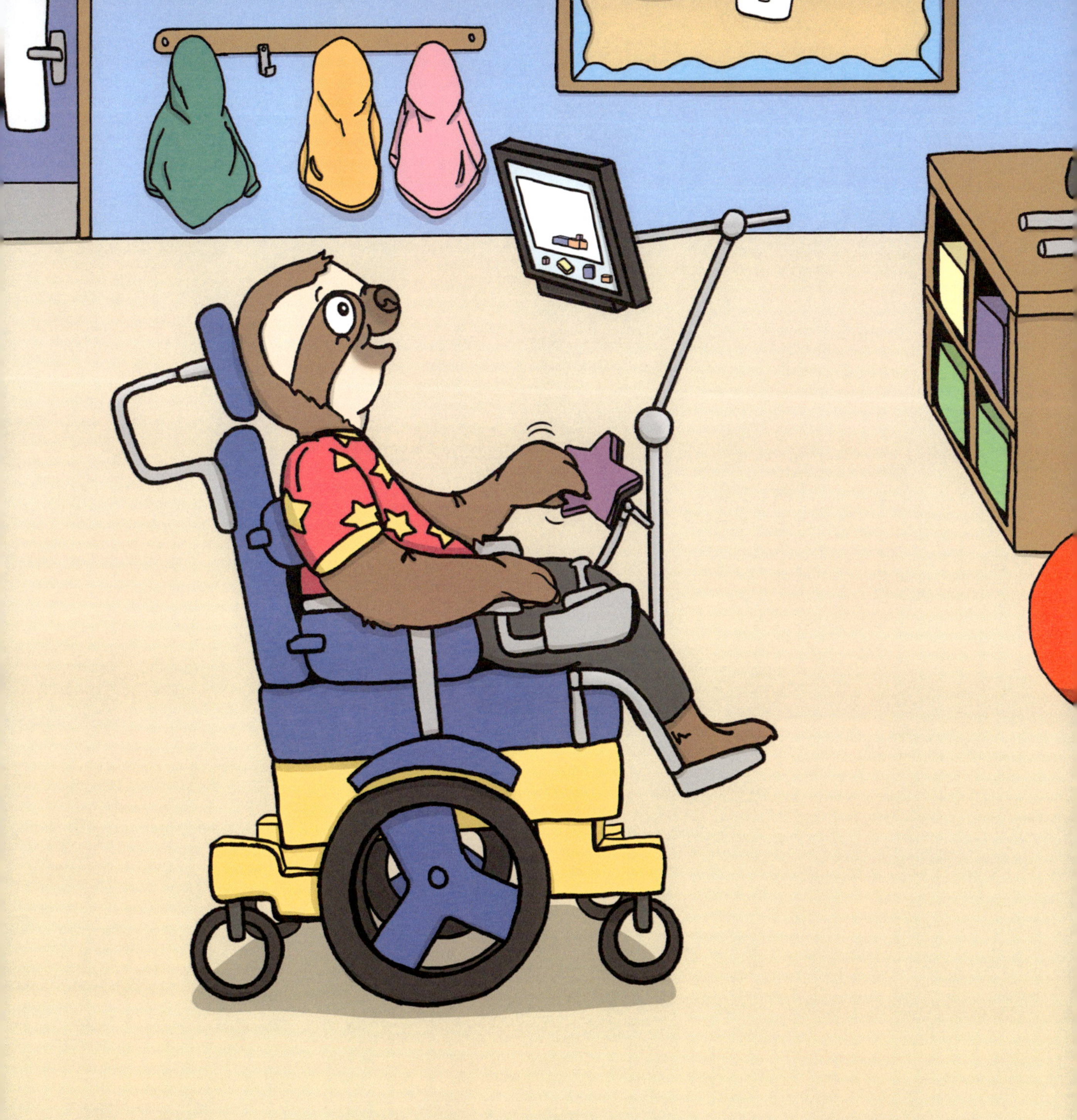

Now it's time for lessons

And all of us can see

That Syed used switches

In lessons one, two and three

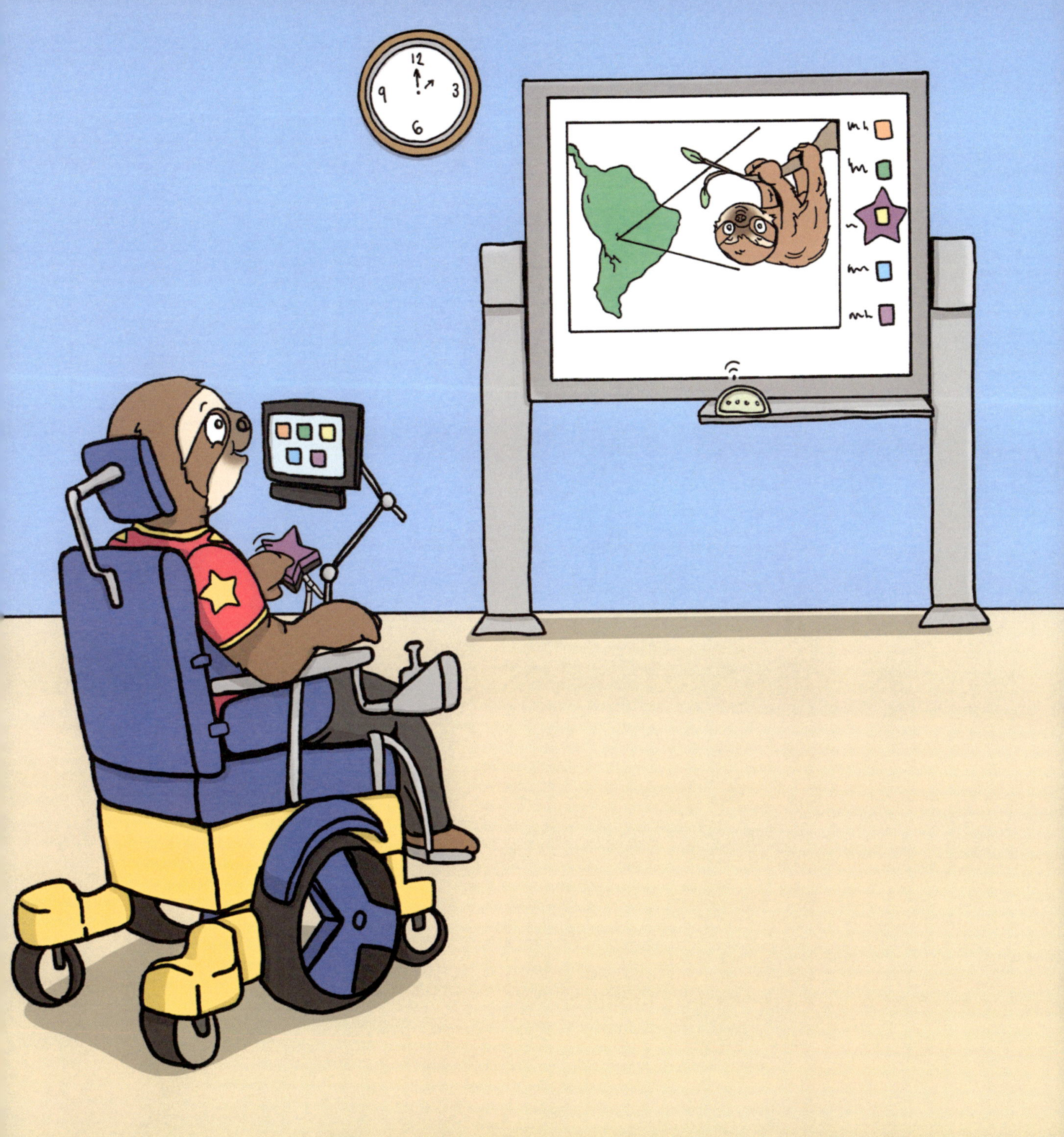

His switches give
him leisure time

To talk and to write

He uses them to drive his chair

Turn on and off the light

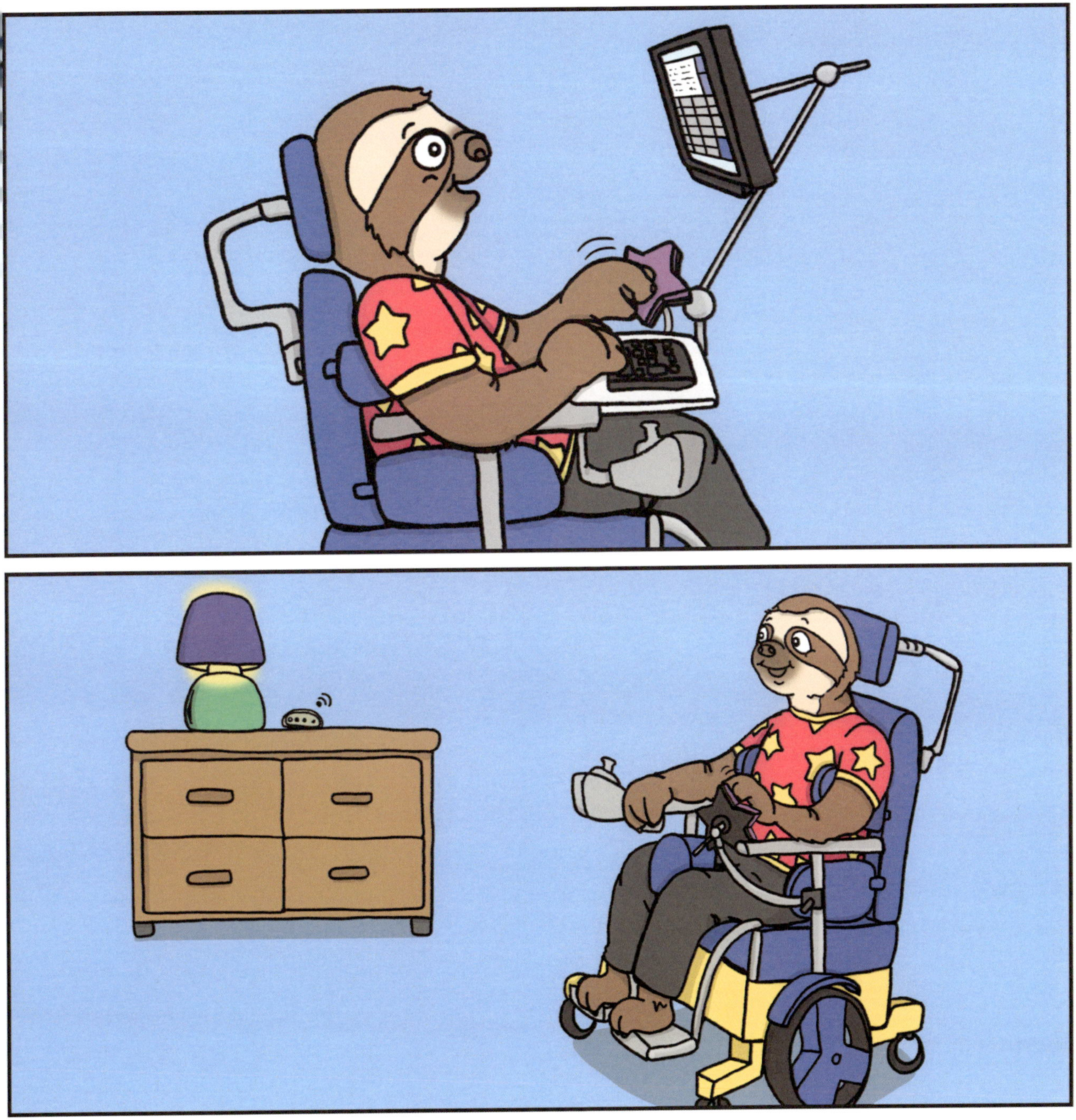

He uses switches all the time

To access school and home

This puts him in full control

To do things on his own

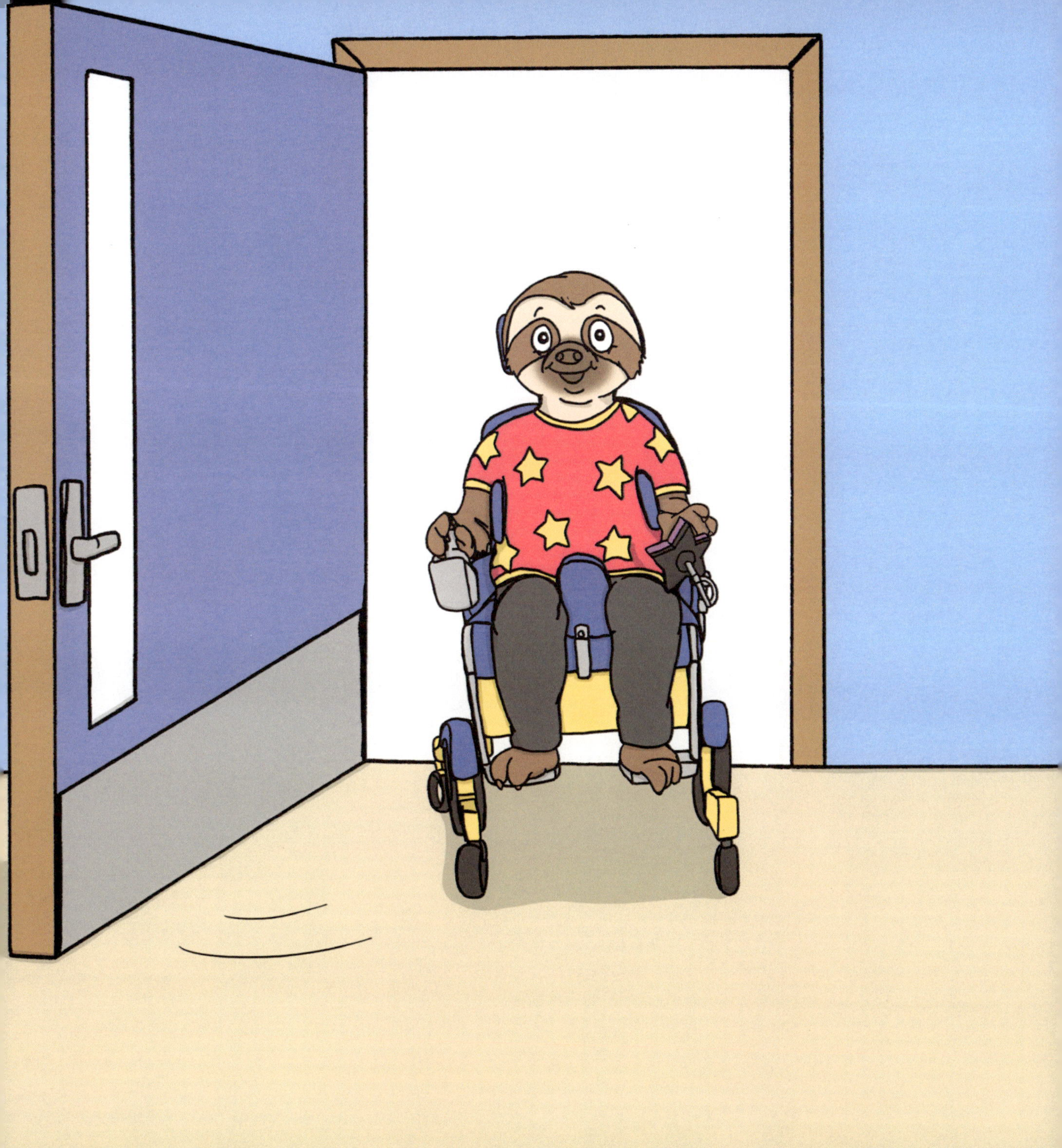

Syed is a switch hero!

His button is a purple star

You are now a super user

A switch hero is what you are!

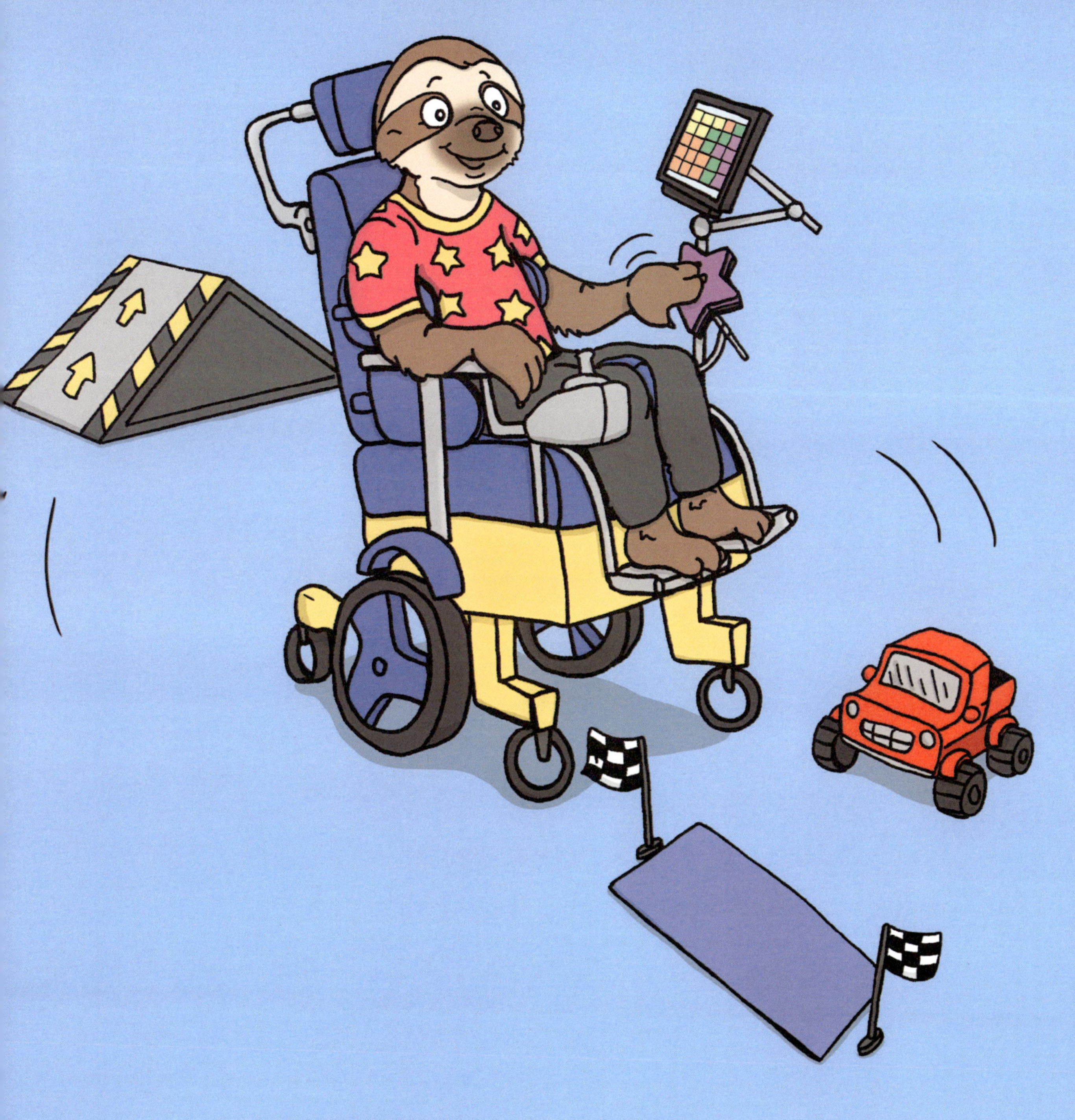

You can use your switches

For so many different things

From games and schoolwork
to self-care

The independence that
it brings!

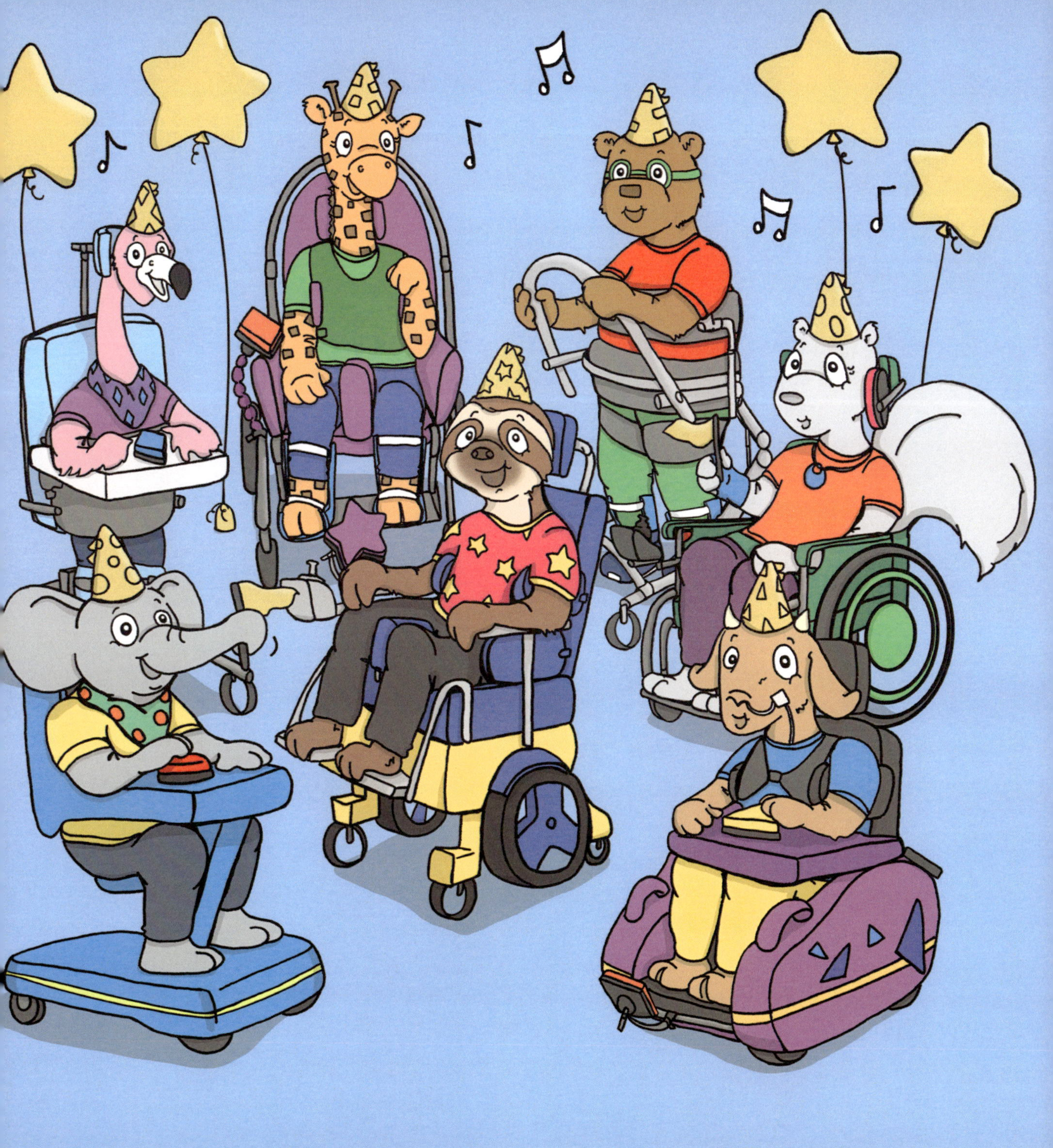

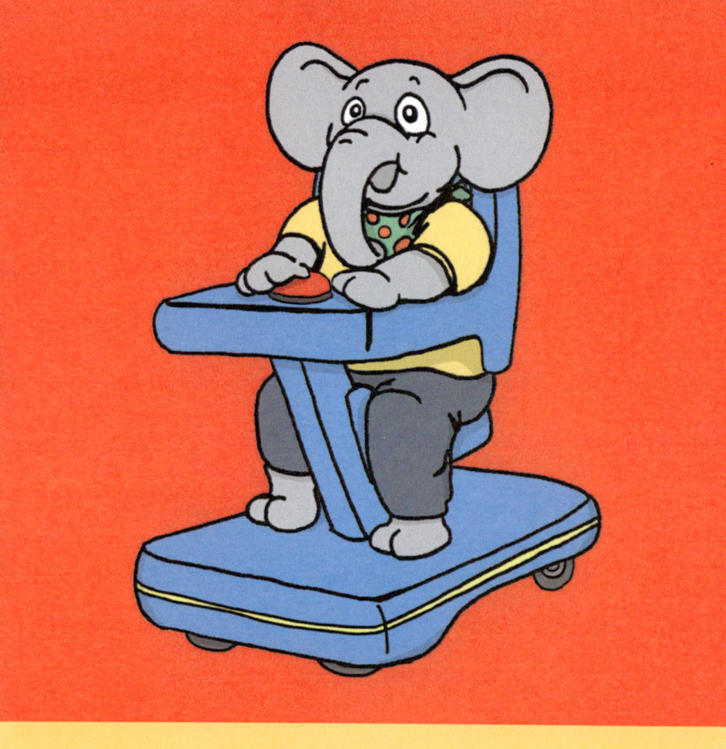

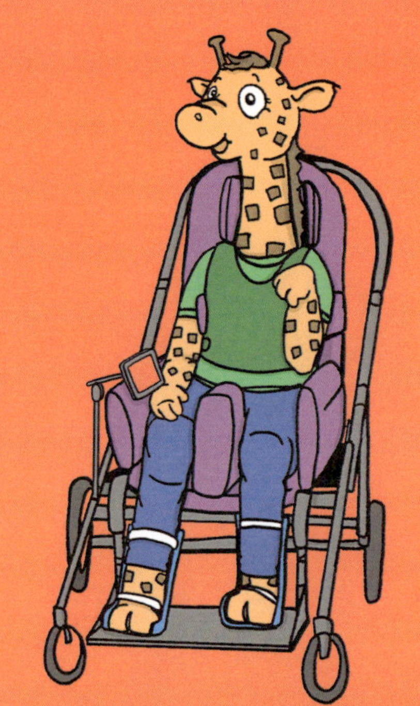

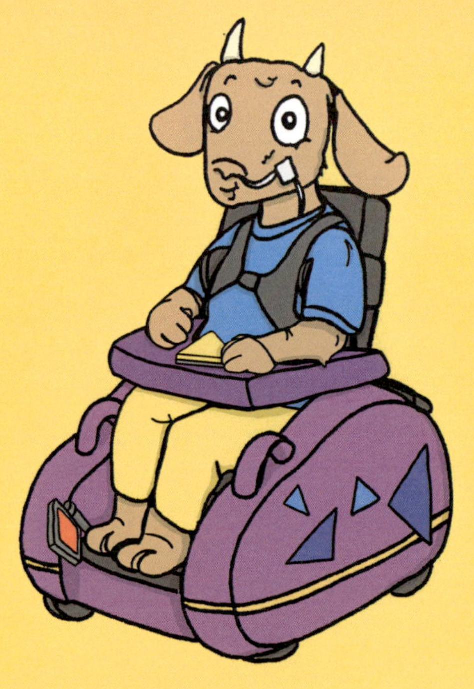

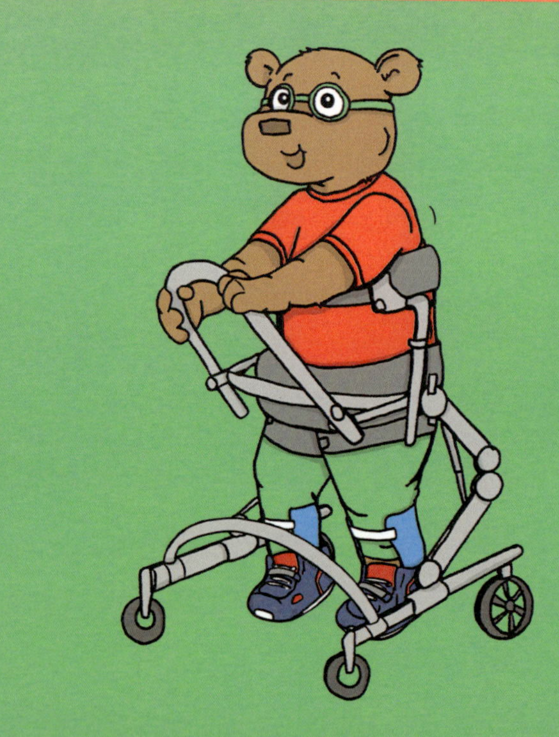

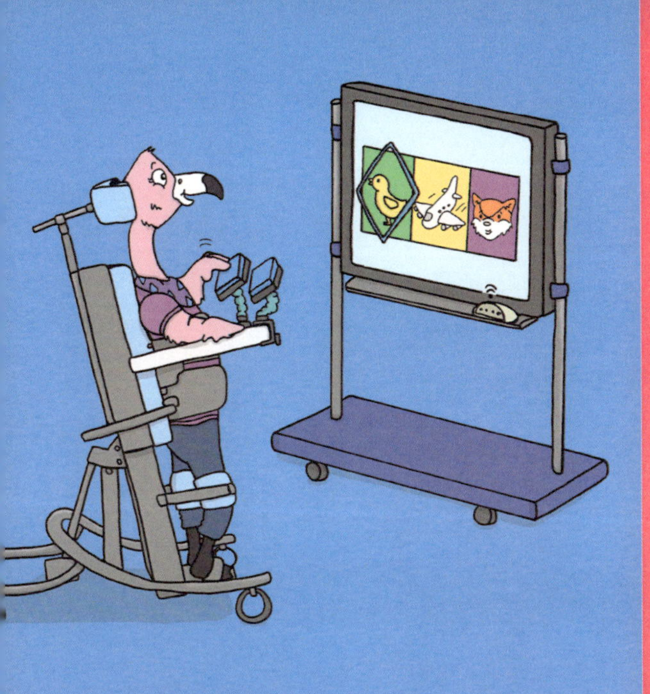

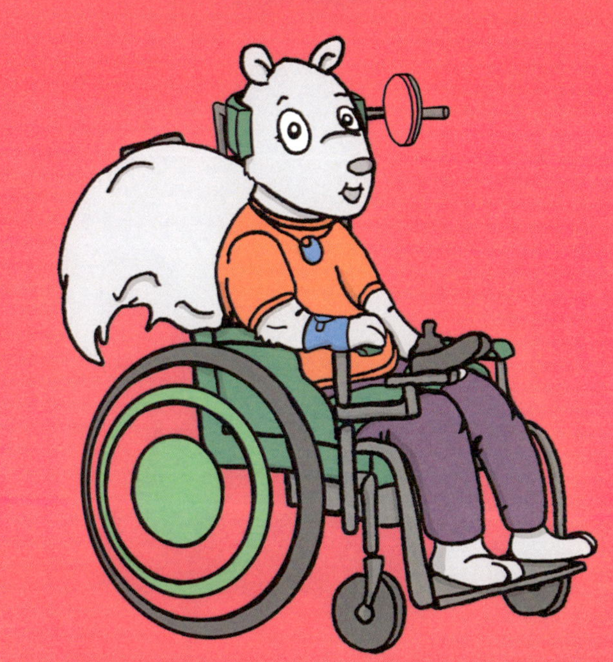

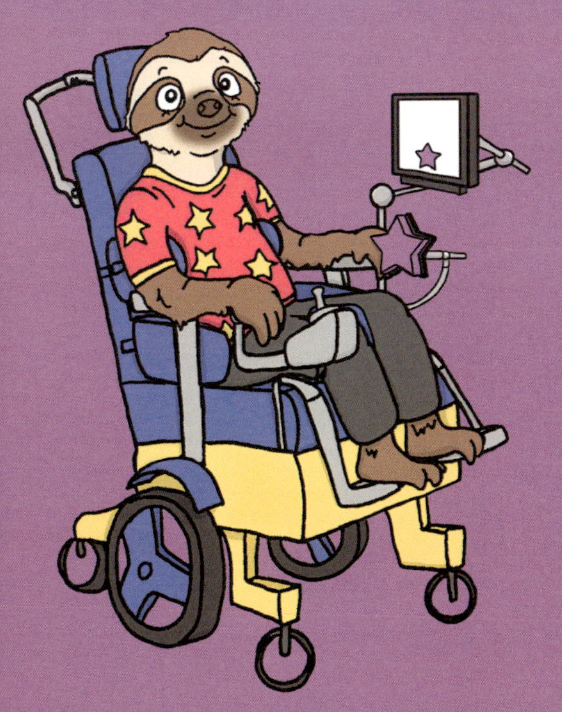

Photo of you!

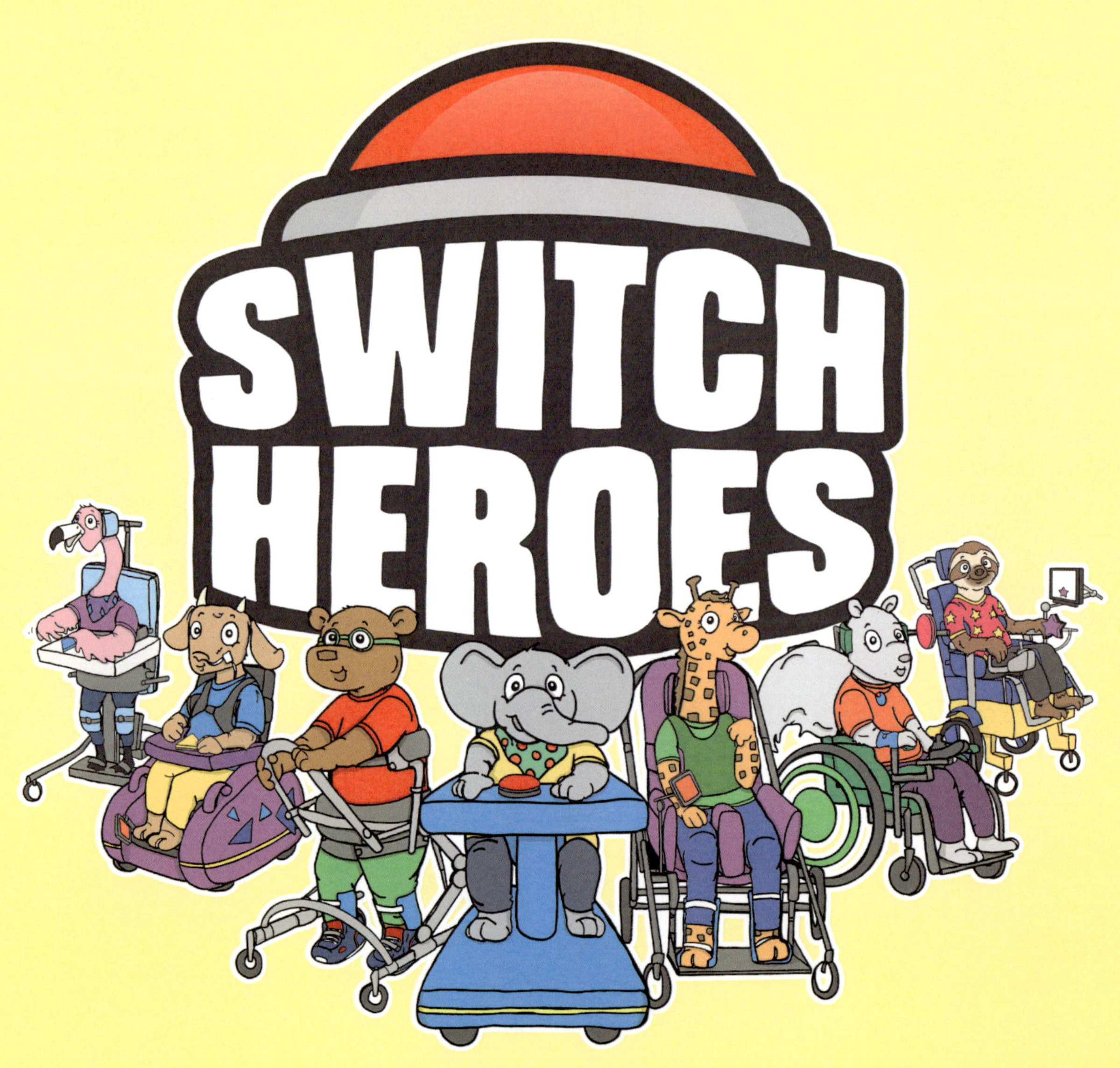
SWITCH
HEROES

The Seven Stages of Switch Development

The Seven Stages of Switch Development is a resource designed for switch-users, their families, caregivers and those who assist them in using switches. It features child-friendly characters and stories that support everyones learning.

The framework provides a helpful reference for measuring and tracking progress while offering flexibility to accommodate the unique needs and preferences of each switch-user.

Written directly to the switch-user, the framework can be read to them if they are unable to read it themselves. Our aim is to ensure that those supporting the child/switch-user can prioritise the child's needs and perspective in the process of developing their switch skills. We have seen the impact of involving the child in the learning process. Seeking their input and feedback regularly empowers them to take an active role in their development and combat learned helplessness.

Adapted from: Bean, I. (2011). Switch Progression Learning Journeys Road Map. Inclusive Technology.
Burkhart, L. (2018). Stepping Stones to Switch Access. Perspectives of the ASHA Special Interest Groups, 3(12), pp.33-44. doi:https://doi/10.1044/persp3.sig12.33.

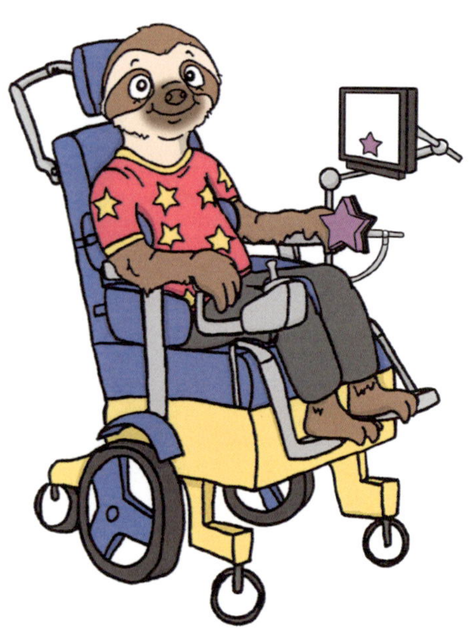

Stage 7

Independent in functional use

Celebrating Syed the Sloth

Star/Purple

Definition

Celebrating Syed is the stage where you will learn to use switches to functionally control multiple software and devices across your day. For example, you can use switches for communication using an AAC device, powered mobility, gaming, browsing the internet, writing and so much more. You will learn how to easily navigate between these different devices and software as well as being able to adjust the settings.

Milestones

- You've mastered switches, using them accurately and consistently
- You can apply your switch skills across different software and devices
- You actively use switches for communication, gaming, browsing, and more
- You're versatile, using switches at home, school, and in the community
- You troubleshoot any switch issues, making necessary adjustments with confidence
- You're a strong advocate, effectively communicating your switch needs to others

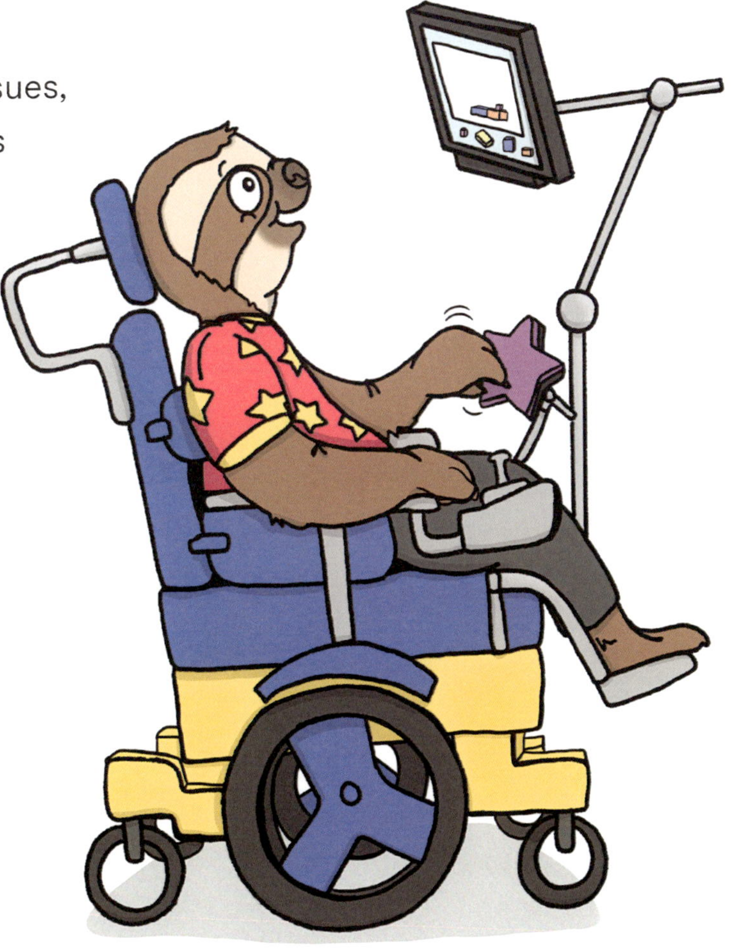

Top tips

- Keep things interesting for the switch-user to maintain their motivation to use switches
- Consider mounting options to ensure their switches are always available on all of their mobility equipment
- Encourage the user to use switches in a variety of settings and situations
- Provide opportunities for the user to practice using switches independently
- Encourage problem-solving and self-determination by allowing the user to choose activities and tasks that they are interested in and can successfully complete using switches
- Ensure you regularly ask for the switch-user's opinion on their switches and software and adapt the requirements based on their ideas and preferences
- Continue to set goals around the switch-user's future independence and how they can progress further based on their own interests and aspirations

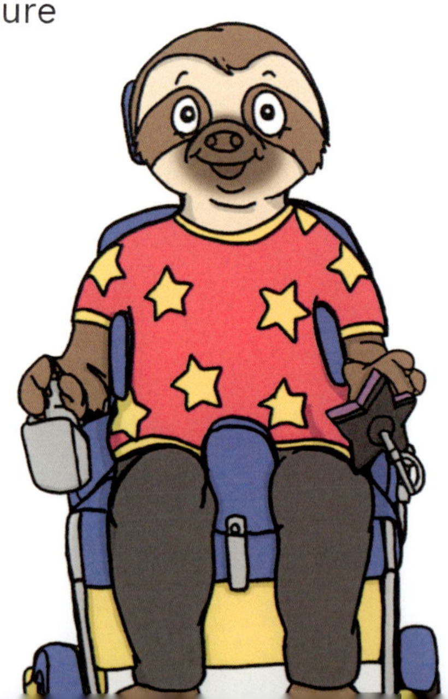

Activities

- Provide opportunities to develop literacy skills through using a keyboard and spelling
- Explore communication software powered by high-tech Augmentative and Alternative Communication (AAC) solutions
- Computer access: Using switches to access and navigate a computer independently, such as typing or browsing the internet
- Environmental control: Using switches to control elements in the environment, such as turning on lights or adjusting the temperature
- Leisure activities: Using switches to engage in leisure activities independently, such as playing games, listening to music, or watching videos

Instead of a prompt hierarchy where the type of prompt increase in support level, we recommend our one prompt switch support cycle. Find out more at Jiao.life

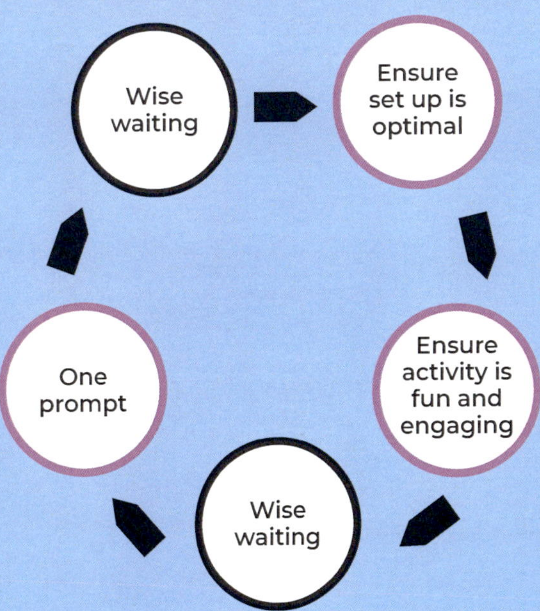

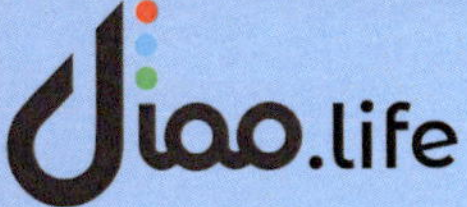

The Assessment Tool

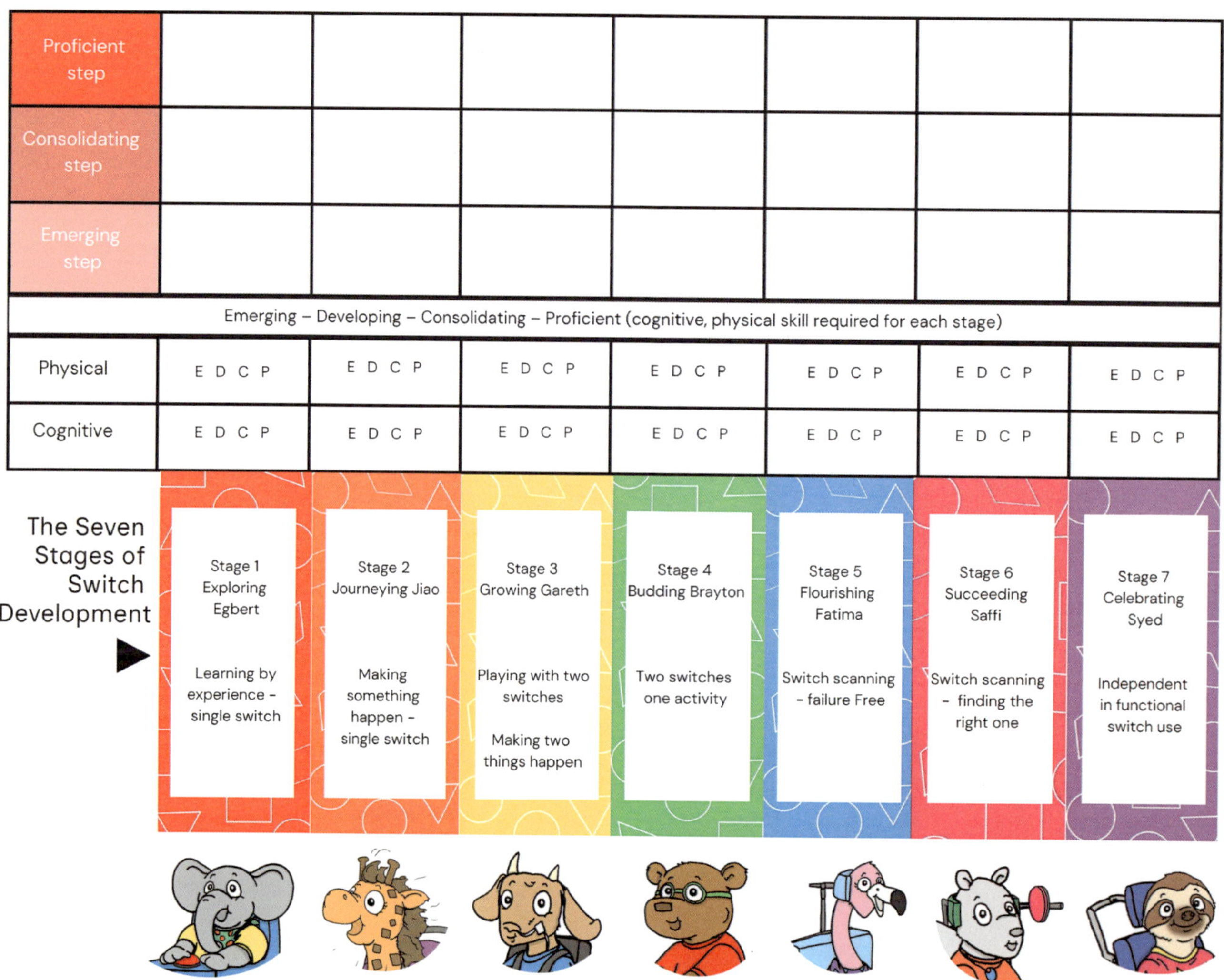

Proficient step							
Consolidating step							
Emerging step							
Emerging – Developing – Consolidating – Proficient (cognitive, physical skill required for each stage)							
Physical	E D C P	E D C P	E D C P	E D C P	E D C P	E D C P	E D C P
Cognitive	E D C P	E D C P	E D C P	E D C P	E D C P	E D C P	E D C P
The Seven Stages of Switch Development ▶	Stage 1 Exploring Egbert Learning by experience - single switch	Stage 2 Journeying Jiao Making something happen - single switch	Stage 3 Growing Gareth Playing with two switches Making two things happen	Stage 4 Budding Brayton Two switches one activity	Stage 5 Flourishing Fatima Switch scanning - failure Free	Stage 6 Succeeding Saffi Switch scanning - finding the right one	Stage 7 Celebrating Syed Independent in functional switch use

Print version available at jiao.life

How to use the assessment tool

- The stages of switch development are not mutually exclusive, so progress can be made across multiple stages simultaneously
- Once a step is completed, mark it off and add the date
- The assessment tool can be used for goal setting, where helpers can add target dates and change the text/box colour accordingly
- There is a stream for assessing cognitive and physical skill development, divided into four steps for each stage (Emerging, Developing, Consolidating and Proficient)
- Helpers should consider the cognitive and physical skills required for each level
- This additional stream can help identify areas that may require additional support and highlight strengths and weaknesses for targeted interventions

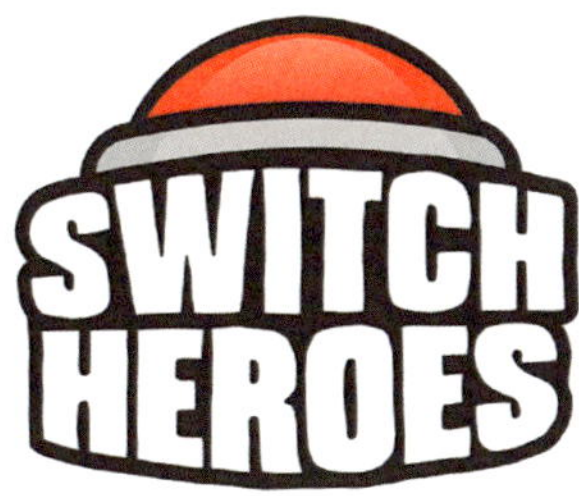

At Jiao Ltd, we are dedicated to empowering individuals through innovative assistive technology solutions.

We provide personalised services and training to help children, families, and professionals navigate the world of assistive tech. For more resources, training options, or to learn how we can support you, visit Jiao.life or get in touch with us directly. We look forward to hearing from you!

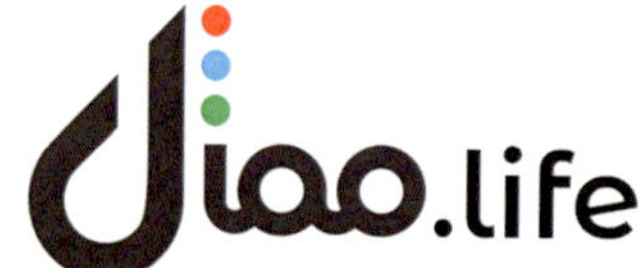

This is to certify that

____

is an independant
switch user

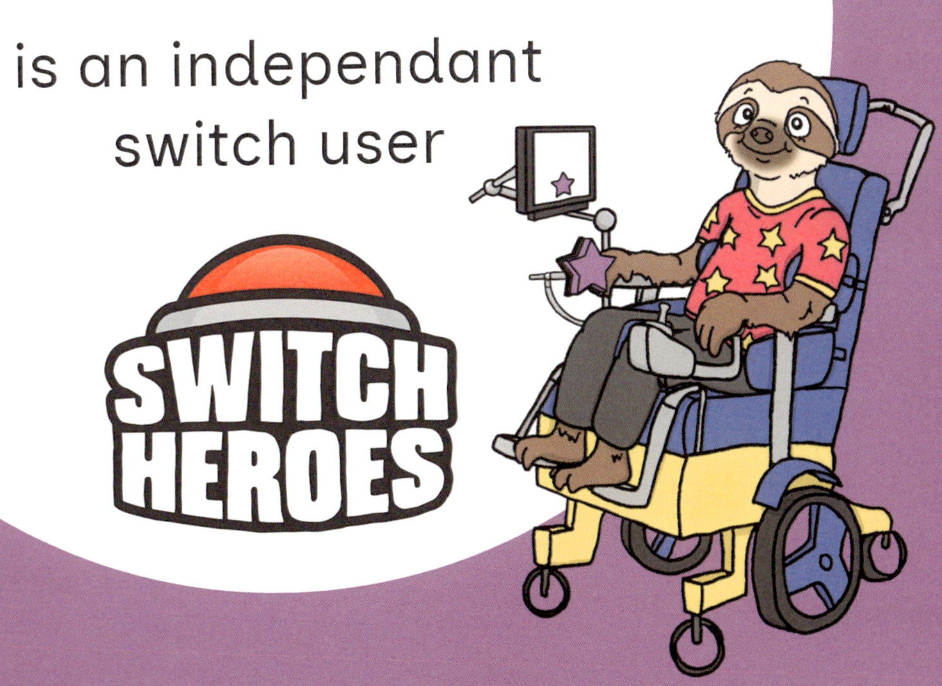

Notes

www.ingramcontent.com/pod-product-compliance
Ingram Content Group UK Ltd.
Pitfield, Milton Keynes, MK11 3LW, UK
UKRC032027290726
14090UKWH00008B/482